The Effectiveness of Acupuncture

Table of contents:

- Introduction
- Audit
- Measuring Outcomes
- Results
- Top Five Best Results
- Excellent Responders
- Non-Responders
- Results of Different Injection Therapies
- Paediatrics
- Other Audits
- Smoking
- Conclusion
- About Author

Introduction:

This is an audit of 784 patients having received acupuncture treatment in a Physical Medicine & Rehabilitation Clinic of a private hospital in İstanbul between June 2017-September 2019. The mean age of patients was 40.6 (SD:13.1- range 9-89 years). 72% were women, with a ratio of 2.6/1 women to men. There were 17 child patients (<18 years). The mean number of acupuncture sessions were 4.3 (Standard deviation-SD 2.3). The first three sessions were completed every three days, and the remaining sessions once a week. Patients received Electroacupuncture most of the time, and occasionally manual acupuncture.

Many patients received acupuncture treatment for more than one diagnosis and multiple body parts, so all evaluations and outcomes were determined for the total number of treatments/cases which were 1091 treatments. For example, if the patient received acupuncture treatment for back, knee and insomnia; it was counted as 3 patients/treatments with each outcome considered separate.

There were a total of 46 diagnosis, but then related diagnosis and body parts were grouped as in 10 main parts, and remaining small groups accumulated as in category 'others'. The groups were;

1. Back pain (215 treatments, 19.7%),
2. Neck pain (196 treatments, 18%),
3. Dorsal strain, including also costo-chondral pain, trigger points, and scoliosis (139 treatments, 12.7%),
4. Fibromyalgia and anxiety disorders (93 treatments, 8.5%),
5. Shoulder pain (86 treatments, 7.9%),
6. Obesity (75 treatments, 6.9%),
7. Migraine and tension headache (49 treatments, 4.5%),
8. Ankle-foot pain, and epin calcanei-heel spur (49 treatments, 4.5%),
9. Knee pain (47 treatments, 4.3%),
10. Calf pain with trigger point in Gastrocnemius (32 treatments, 2.9%),

11. Others (110 treatments, 10.1%). This group includes various diagnosis such as bell's palsy, hip pain, sacroiliac dysfunction, coccyx pain, lateral epicondylitis, cessation of smoking, nausea, multiple sclerosis, vertigo, restless leg syndrome, polyneuropathy.

Mean duration of pain was 31 months (Standard Deviation 47.5). In the 'smoking cessation' group, mean time of smoking was 167 months, so being a longer duration, that was counted separately.

Measuring Outcomes: Patients were asked to score their pain level on a VAS (Visual Analogue Scale) before the start of the first treatment session. After 3-4 days from the end of acupuncture sessions, their level of pain was recorded again on a VAS, and from the difference of VAS, a percentage improvement was calculated. The percentages were than grouped as:

1-nil: no improvement,

2-minimal: 1-32% improvement,

3-moderate: 33-50% improvement,

4-good: 51-80% improvement

5-excellent: 81-100% improvement.

Therefore >50% =good+excellent.

and >33% =moderate+good+excellent.

The outcomes for 1091 treatments (cases-treated patients) were:

10 % (109 treatments) nil-no improvement;

13% (141) minimal improvement;

5% (52) moderate;

41% (449) good;

31% (336) excellent.

The success rate was established as a range of 'excellent+good' to excellent+good+moderate improvement'. So, the overall success rate was **72-77%.**

 The success rates for the main 10 diagnosis were found as follows:

1-For back pain the success rate was 72%-64%.

2-Neck pain: **83%-78%**

3-Dorsal strain: 77%-66%

4-Fibromyalgia and anxiety disorders: **83%-80%**

5-Shoulder pain :79%-78%

6-Obesity: 63%-61%

7-Migraine and tension headache: **86%-82%**

8-Ankle sprains/foot pain and heel spur: 80 %

9- Knee pain: **87-81%**

10-Calf pain and trigger point in Gastrocnemius 75-81%

Others: 75-86%

Including also the smallest groups (together with the one inside the group 'others') the conditions/diagnosis showing highest percentage of **'excellent improvement'** were: Bell's palsy: 70% of patients with Bell's palsy; 60% of patients treated for cessation of smoking, 67% of vertigo patients;

67% inflammatory bowel disease patients; and 53% of ankle pain patients showed excellent improvement.

Evaluating the child patients (<18 years); the main diagnosis of treatment was for obesity (41%) having a success rate of 45% (excellent+good), while in the obese adult group was 68%.

Another evaluation was made for the patients having received other injections such as Neural therapy, Intra-articular Hyaluronic Acid (HA) and Acupuncture consecutively. In 15 patients acupuncture showed better improvement than

Neural therapy, in 6 patients acupuncture better than HA, whereas in 6 patients Neural therapy was more successful than acupuncture.

Side effects: No serious side effects were seen except vasovagal syncope in one patient, bruising, and forgotten needles among the hair in 5 patients which didn't cause serious problem.

In conclusion: This audit includes a large variety of patients predominantly musculoskeletal pain. In this group of acupuncture patient's high success rates were obtained compared to General Practitioner results, which can be due to the appropriate selection of patients and the fact that PMR clinic is a more specialized one. The audit allowed me to identify the categories which acupuncture achieved the greatest success rates thus enabling me to advise my patients regarding optimal treatment options.

An Audit of the Effectiveness of Acupuncture in a Physical Medicine Rehabilitation Clinic

Dr. Evren Kul Panza

- This is an audit of <u>784 patients</u> having received acupuncture treatment.

- Many patients received acupuncture treatment for more than one diagnosis and <u>multiple body parts</u>,

- Therefore all evaluations and outcomes were determined for the total number of cases which were <u>1091 cases/patients.</u>

- For example, if the patient received acupuncture treatment for back, knee and insomnia; it was counted as 3 cases with each outcome considered separate.

- They were the patients who applied to Physical Medicine & Rehabilitation clinic of the private hospital where I work.

- Between June 2017-September 2019.

- All data was analyzed retrospectively.

- The mean age of patients was 40.6 (SD:13.1-
  range 9-89 years).

- 72% were women and 28% men, with a ratio of 2.6/1 women to men.

- There were 17 child patients (<18 years).

- The mean number of acupuncture sessions were 4.3
  (-SD 2.3).
  in men it was 4.1, and in women : 4.5

*SD = Standard Deviation – a quantity expressing by how much the members of a group differ from the mean (average) value for the group

Gender distribution among patients

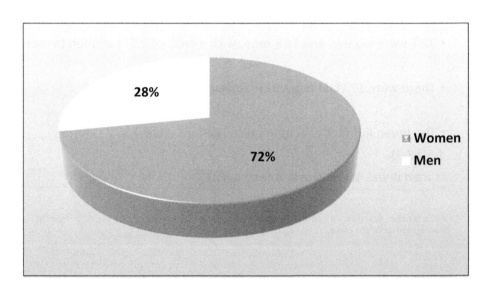

- There were 9 patients as drop-outs.

- They were defined as those who did not attend the controls and who could not be contacted by phone.

- 7 of them had completed only one session, and 2 had four sessions.

- These drop-outs were not counted in the statistics and were left out of the audit.

- Therefore the audit involved **784 patients**, and considering multiple treatments **1091 cases.**

- Mean duration of pain and symptoms was 31 months. (Standard deviation 47.5)

- In the 'smoking cessation' group, which had 10 patients, mean duration of smoking was 167 months, so not to influence the mean, that was counted separately.

Acupuncture was applied for 46 different diagnosis.

Name of Diagnosis	Number of cases/patients
1-Cervical strain	136
2-Dorsal strain	115
3-Lumbar hernia	97
4-Shoulder pain	86
5-Lumbar radiculopathy	80
6-Obesity	75
7-Fibromyalgia	60
8-Cervical hernia	60
9-Knee pain	47
10-Migraine	38
11-Calf pain-GC trigger point	32
12-Ankle pain	28
13-Hip pain	22
14-Lumbar strain	21
15-Lateral epicondylitis	16
16-Heel spur	15

Name of Diagnosis	Number of cases/patients
17-Scoliosis	14
18-Hand-wrist pain	14
19-Tension type headache	11
20-Chest pain/costochondritis	10
21-Facial pain	10
22-Smoking sessation	10
23-Failed-back surgery	9
24-Panic attack	9
25-Depression	9
26-İnsomnia	9
27-Sacroiliac dysfunction	8
28-Bell's palsy	7
29-Anxiety	6
30-Foot pain	6

Name of Diagnosis	Number of cases/patients
31-Operation on the face	3
32-Inflammatory bowel disease	3
33-Coccydinia	3
34-Hemiparesis	3
35-Vertigo	3
36-Asthma	2
37-Carpal tunnel syndrome	2
38-Postmenopausal symptoms	2
39-Multiple sclerosis	2
40-Nausea	2
41-Polyneuropathy	2
42-Allergy	1
43-ALS	1
44-Dementia	1
45-Restless leg syndrome	1
46-Trigeminal neuralgia	1

All 46 Diagnosis

Diagnosis Number

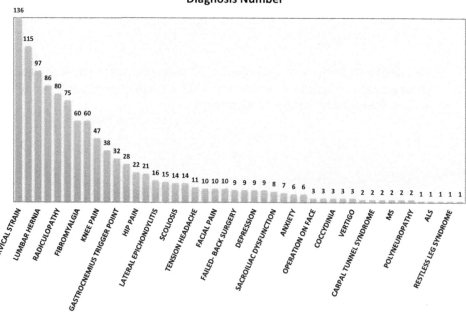

- In order to have more visible results, all diagnosis were gathered and grouped into 10 main parts, and remaining small groups were accumulated in the category '*Others*'.

MAIN DIAGNOSIS GROUPS

- 1 Back pain (215 cases, 19.7%),

- 2 Neck pain (196 cases, 18%),

- 3 Dorsal strain, including also costochondritis , trigger points, and scoliosis (139 cases, 12.7%),

- 4 Fibromyalgia and anxiety disorders (93 cases, 8.5%),

- 5 Shoulder pain (86 cases, 7.9%),

- 6 Obesity (75 cases, 6.9%),

- 7 Migraine and tension headache (49 cases, 4.5%),

- 8 Ankle-foot pain, and heel spur (49 cases, 4.5%),

- 9 Knee pain (47 cases, 4.3%),

- 10 Calf pain with trigger point in Gastrocnemius (32 cases, 2.9%)

- 11 Others (110 cases, 10.1%).

Distribution of cases according to main diagnosis groups

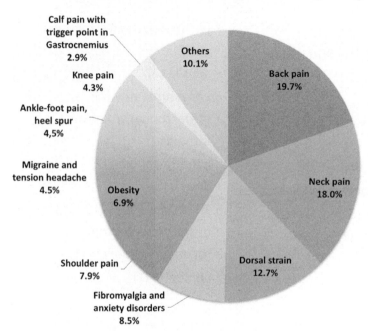

23

The group defined as <u>'Others'</u>

- hip pain (22 cases),
- lateral epicondylitis(16 cases),
- wrist pain (12)
- smoking (10),
- facial pain (9),
- Bell's palsy (7)
- operation on the face (3)
- inflammatory bowel disease (3),
- coccydynia (3),
- hemiparesis (3),
- vertigo(3),
- postmenopausal symptoms(2),
- ms (2),
- nausea (2),
- polyneuropathy (2),
- carpal tunnel syndrome (2),
- asthma (2),
- hand-finger pain (2)
- allergy (1),
- als (1),
- restless leg syndrome (1),
- trigeminal neuralgia (1),
- dementia (1)

Application of Acupuncture (AP) Sessions

- Manual AP and Electroacupuncture were applied.

- Seirin disposable needles were used.

- EA was applied as intermittent 2/15 Hz.

- Sessions lasted 20-30 minutes.

- In general, first 4 sessions were applied every 3 days, and the following sessions once a week, but this could change according to the patient.

- Patients were called 3-4 days after the last AP session for control assessment.

- In case they didn't come in further days, they were phoned by my assistant and asked about VAS for pain.

Measuring Outcomes:

VAS

- Their pain level was scored on a **VAS** before the start of the first session.

- After 3-4 days from the end of acupuncture sessions, level of pain was recorded again on **VAS**,

- <u>**From the difference of VAS, a percentage of improvement was calculated.**</u>

The percentages of improvement according to decrease in VAS were then grouped as:

- *1-nil*: no improvement,
- *2-minimal(poor)*: 1-30% improvement,
- *3-moderate*: 31-50% improvement,
- *4-good:* 51-80% improvement
- *5-excellent:* 81-100% improvement.

Classification of obesity outcomes

- In case patient loses >10% of her/his weight ➔ excellent improvement
- If the patient loses 5-10% of her/his weight ➔ good improvement
- If loses 3%-5% of her weight ➔ moderate
- İf loses 0-3% ➔ poor improvement

Defining outcomes for cessation of smoking

- If the patient quits smoking totally➔ defined as 'excellent'

- If the number of cigarettes daily drops by 80% ➔ 'good improvement'

- If the number drops by 50%-80% ➔ ' moderate improvement'

- If drops by 0-50% ➔ poor improvement.

The outcomes for 1091 cases :

- **10 %** (109 cases) no improvement/non-responsive

- **13%** (141)minimal/poor improvement(meaning 1-30%)

- **5%** (52) moderate improvement (meaning 31-50%)

- **41%** (449) good improvement(meaning 51-80%)

- **31%** (336) excellent improvement(meaning 81-100%)

RESULTS

	Number of cases	%
Nil-no improvement (0%)	109	10%
Poor-minimal improvement (1-30%)	141	13%
Moderate improvement (31-50%)	52	5%
Good improvement (51-80%)	449	41%
Excellent improvement (81-100%)	336	31%
TOTAL	1091	100%

Success rate

- The success rate was established as a range of 'excellent+good' to excellent+good+moderate improvement'.

- So the overall success rate was 72-77%.

- The small difference may be due to the relatively narrow range of 'moderate group' which I defined as 31%-50% improvement.

- Therefore when I wanted to summarize as a single value, most of the times I defined the success rate as only 'good+excellent' improvement.

- Which corresponded to >51% improvement (51%-80% plus 81%-100%)

Overall Success rate of 1091 cases as 'excellent+good improvement' was : 72%

**In women : 73%
**In men : 71.7%

The success rates for the main 10 diagnosis

- 1-For back pain the success rate was 64%-72%.
- 2-*Neck pain* : **78%-83%**
- 3-Dorsal strain : 66%-77%
- 4-*Fibromyalgia and anxiety disorders* : **80%-83%**
- 5-Shoulder pain : 78%-79%
- 6-Obesity: 61%-63%
- 7-*Migraine and tension headache* : **82%-86%**
- 8- *Ankle sprains/foot pain and heel spur*: **80%-80 %**
- 9- *Knee pain*: **81%-87%**
- 10-Calf pain and trigger point in Gastrocnemius 75%-81%
- 11-Others: **75%-86%**

Success rates as 'good+ excellent improvement'

Diagnosis	Success rates (good+excellent improvement)
Migraine and tension type headaches	82%
Knee pain	81%
Fibromyalgia and anxiety disorders	80%
Ankle pain-sprains/foot pain and heel spur	80%
Neck pain	78%
Shoulder pain	78%
Calf pain/ trigger point in Gastrocnemius	75%
Others	75%
Dorsal strain	66%
Back pain	64%
Obesity	61%

Success Rates (as excellent+good)

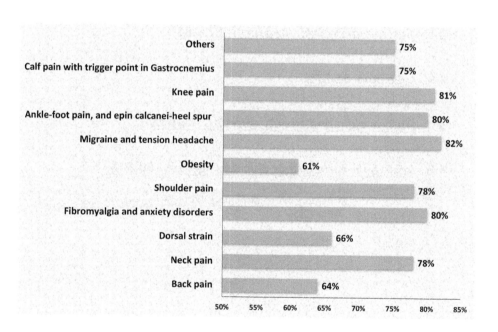

Top 5 best results:

- 1st: _Migraine and tension headache_ **82%-86%**

- 2nd: _Knee pain_ **81-87%**

- 3rd : _Fibromyalgia and anxiety disorders_ **80-83%**

- 4th : _Ankle pain-sprains/foot pain and heel spur_ **80-80%**

- 5th : _Neck pain_ **78%-88%**

Top 5 categories in terms of best outcome'

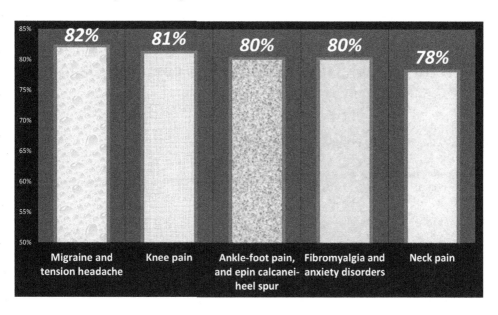

The group 'Others'- other less common diagnosis):

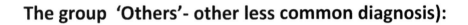

• 110 cases, 10.1% of all.(110/1091)

• Success rate was 75-86%

'Others'

- hip pain (22 cases),
- lateral epicondylitis (16 cases),
- wrist pain (12)
- smoking (10),
- facial pain (9),
- bell's palsy (7)
- operation on the face (3)
- inflammatory bowel disease (3),
- coccydynia (3),
- hemiparesis(3),
- vertigo(3),
- *postmenopausal* symptoms(2),
- ms (2),
- nausea (2),
- polyneuropathy (2),
- carpal tunnel syndrome (2),
- asthma (2),
- hand-finger pain (2)
- allergy (1),
- als (1),
- restless leg syndrome (1),
- trigeminal neuralgia (1),
- dementia (1)

Including the small groups as well,
(ALL 46 diagnosis).

Which conditions/diagnosis
showed highest percentage of
'excellent improvement' (81-100%)?

'Excellent improvement'
improvement of 81-100%
(including all 46 diagnosis)

- 70% of patients with Bell's palsy; (7 out of 10),
- 67% of *vertigo* ; (2 out of 3)
- 67 % *inflammatory bowel disease*;(2 out of 3)
- 60% of patients treated for *cessation of smoking*, (6 out of 10)
- 58% of *migraine* (22 out of 38)
- 53% of *ankle pain* (15 out of 29)
- 44 % of *depression* (4 out of 9)

The 'Excellent outcome '(81-100%) (among all 46 diagnois)

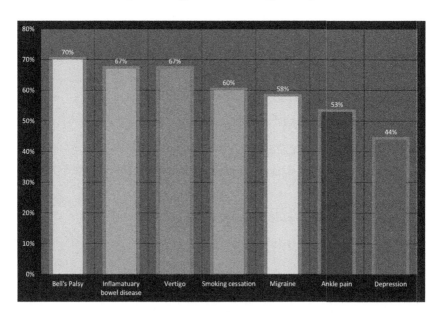

Non responsive group
= 'No improvement'

- The patients who didn't heal at all.
- 110 cases.
- mean age of this group was 41.4
- mean duration of pain was 33.2 months.
   * in overall group was 31.
- Mean number of sessions was 4.3

- Women/men ratio in 'non responsive' group was 75%-25%
- While in the overall was 72%-28%

- Which means <u>among the non responsive patients, women were relatively more than men.</u>

Non responsive group

	Number of patients	Percentage(%)
Back pain	27	24.5%
Dorsal pain	17	15.5%
Others	16	14.5%
Obesity	13	11.8%
Neck pain	10	9.1%
Fibromyalgia and anxiety disorders	10	9.1%
Shoulder pain	7	6.4%
Knee pain	4	3.6%
Migraine and tension headache	3	2.7%
Calf pain &trigger point in Gastrocnemius	2	1.8%
Foot/ankle pain& heel spur	1	0.9%

Distribution of diagnosis in 'non responsive' group

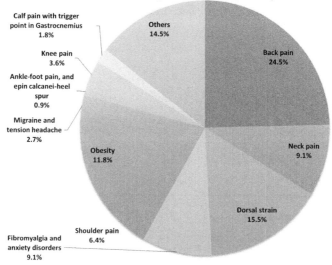

Calf pain with trigger point in Gastrocnemius 1.8%

Knee pain 3.6%

Ankle-foot pain, and epin calcanei-heel spur 0.9%

Migraine and tension headache 2.7%

Obesity 11.8%

Fibromyalgia and anxiety disorders 9.1%

Shoulder pain 6.4%

Others 14.5%

Back pain 24.5%

Neck pain 9.1%

Dorsal strain 15.5%

Comparison

Distribution of cases/diagnosis among <u>main categories</u>

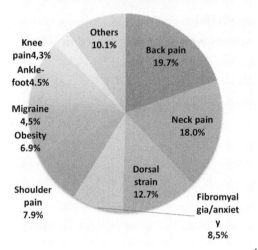

Distribution of cases/diagnosis in <u>'non responsive' group</u>

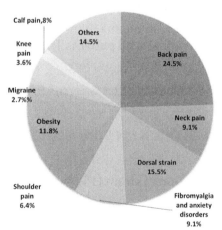

Evaluating the distribution of diagnosis in 'non responsive' group

- Which group of diagnosis had more 'non responsive patients' relatively?

- **1-Back pain patients** (24.5% versus 19.7%)

    (which means there are more patients with back pain who didn't heal considering all patients.)

- **2-Obesity** (11.8% versus 6.9%)

- **3- Others** (14.5 %versus 10.1%)

- **4-Dorsal strain** (15.5% versus 12.7%)

'non responsive' patients received how many AP sessions?

	Number of patients	Percentage (%)
1 session	37	34%
2 sessions	30	27%
3 sessions	23	21%
4 sessions	8	7%
5 sessions	4	4%
6 sessions	5	4.5%
7 sessions	2	1.8%
10 sessions	1	0.9%
Total	110	100%

- Which group of diagnosis had less 'non responsive patients' relatively?

1- Neck pain (9.1% versus 18%)

…which means : considering all category of cases, there are few patients with neck pain who didn't heal.

2- Ankle-foot pain, heel spur (0.9% versus 4.5%)

3- Migraine (2.7% versus 4.5%)

4- Knee pain (3.6% versus 4.3%)

Distribution of number of sessions in "no-improvement" group

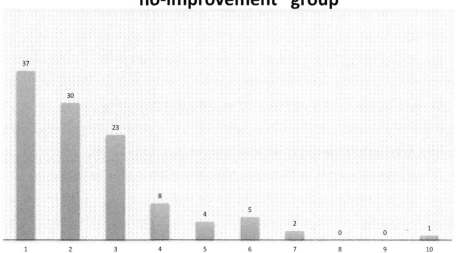

Patients who came Only for 1 session of AP

124 cases (11.3% of 1092) had only one session of AP.

97 were women (78%), 27 men (22%) ➔ W/M **78%-22%**

(the overall distribution of women to men was (72%-28%)
This shows that women had slightly more tendency not to continue.

Outcome of
patients who came only for 1 session

**Excellent improvement : 40.3% (50/124) (in overall was 31%)

**No improvement: 28% (35/124) (in overall was 10%)

Which means:

** 40% of these patients did not continue maybe because they were healed totally,

** however 28% of them didn't continue because they didn't heal at all.

Patients who came for 1 session

- Considering that the mean number of acupuncture <u>sessions was 4 overall, and 31 % had excellent </u>outcome,
- who had <u>just 1 session having a 40% of excellent improvement</u> shows that
- **<u>An optimal result of AP treatment can be achieved even with 1 session sometimes.</u>**
- Considering that also the non-responders are more (28% versus 10%) shows that the outcome in 1 session cases was like 'all or nothing'.

Results of
Different Injection
Therapies

Various injection therapies that I apply

**Acupuncture

**Intraarticular Hyaluronic acid

   -shoulder-subacromial

   -knee

** Neural therapy

  (local/quaddel technique)

   -shoulder-subacromial

   -cervical, dorsal, lumbar paravertebral

(Neural therapy involves injection of Jetocain diluted with saline)

Acupuncture v Neural therapy
&
Acupuncture v Hyaluronic Acid

**in 15 patients : Acupuncture showed better improvement than Neural therapy

**in 6 patients : Neural therapy was more effective than acupuncture.

** in 6 patients (3 knee, 3 shoulder) : acupuncture was more effective than HA

Paediatric patients

- <u>17 patients </u>were under 18 years old.(22% of all cases)
- The youngest patient was 9 years old.
- <u>Their diagnosis were:</u>

- **7 cases obesity**
- **3 cases Bell's palsy**
- **3 cases cervical pain**
- **1 case facial pain**
- **1 case dorsal strain**
- **1 case lumbar strain**

- <u>The overall success rate as 'excellent+good' was 71%</u>
    <u>(in total was 72%)</u>

    7 patients 'excellent',
    5 patients 'good',
    1 patient 'moderate' and
    4 patients 'minimal improvement'

Acupuncture for childhood obesity

- Child patients applied to have AP mainly <u>for obesity</u>
- 7 children out of 17 (41%).

For obesity, losing >5% of body weight was considered good, and >10% was considered excellent.

- The success rate for obesity in the **pediatric patients** (excellent+good) was 45%

- While in **adult obese patients** the success rate was 68%.

- <u>Which means acupuncture works better for adult obesity</u>.
- This may be because the children were not deciding by themselves to have AP, but taken/forced?? ☺ by their parents.

Non Indigenous patients

- 16 patients
- 8 Russian, 2 Ukranian, 2 Italian, 2 Syrian, 1 American, 1 French
- They tended to show a slightly higher improvement
- Success rate was 75%-87.5%
    (compared to 72%-77% in overall)

Maybe because they were more informed about acupuncture.

In the 'Non responsive' group, THE LINK was more EVIDENT

- which proves that if a patient did not respond, it could be because he/she had only 1 or 2 sessions, and didn't continue.

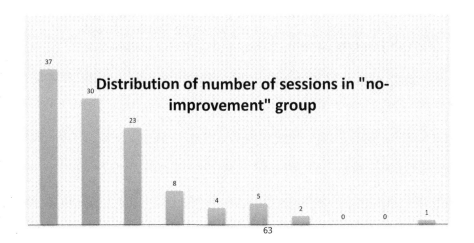

Distribution of number of sessions in "no-improvement" group

37
30
23
8
4
5
2
0
0
1

63

- Being aware of this correlation, increasing number of sessions ➔better outcome.

(even if is not a very strong correlation R:0.35)

- Seeing that <u>improvement was not correlated with age or long duration of symptoms, it</u> is an **encouraging fact for chronic pain and elderly patients** to be candidates for acupuncture.

Correlations According to different diagnosis
in terms of <u>number of AP sessions & Improvement</u>

- 1- Migraine: R: 0.57
- 2- Obesity : R: 0.43
- 3- Shoulder pain: R: 0.40
- 4- Back pain patients: R: 0.32
- 5- Fibromyalgia: R: 0.29
- 6- Neck pain patients: R: 0.26
- 7- Gastrocnemius trigger point-calf pain: R: 0.0

- Which shows that...
- For migraine,
- And for obesity
- better outcomes are obtained with more sessions

- However for calf pain, and trigger point in gastrocnemius, also few sessions are enough.

Distribution of women/men

- Women/Men: 2.6/1.

- This is because clinical pain is reported with higher severity and frequency, longer duration, and present in a greater number of body regions in women than in men.

- Being exposed to repeated painful visceral events (eg menses,labour) during life may contribute to an increased sensitivity to, and greater prevalence of pain among women.**

**Is it All about Sex? Acupuncture for the Treatment of Pain from a Biological and Gender Perspective. Iréne Lund, Thomas Lundeberg

Acupuncture in Medicine, vol. 26, 1: pp. 33-45. , First Published March 1, 2008.

Other audits

- I have not come across audits with large number of cases as in mine.
- The biggest had 500 patients.
- While mine had 784 patients and 1091 cases.

Acupuncture in practice:
mapping the providers, the patients and the
settings in a national cross-sectional survey.
Hopton AK, Curnoe S,Kanaan M, et al. BMJ Open 2012;2:e000456.

- In the <u>survey</u> of Hopton et al. the most common conditions chosen for acupuncture were musculoskeletal diseases as first,
- headache as second;
- depression/anxiety disorders as third.

An Audit of 500 Acupuncture Patients in General Practice
Jonathan Freedman. ACUPUNCTURE IN MEDICINE 2002;20(1):30-34.

In this audit of **500 patients,**

***The most common diagnosis were

*neck pain, *low back pain, *shoulder problems, *hayfever, *knee osteoarthritis, and *migraine.

***Women/men ratio was 3.5/1...in my audit was 2.6/1

***Only manual AP was applied.

*** *overall success rate was 61%(cure)-73% (improvement)*

In my audit *the overall success rate was 72%(good+excellent)-77%(moderate+good+excellent),*

An Audit of 500 Acupuncture Patients in General Practice
Jonathan Freedman. ACUPUNCTURE IN MEDICINE 2002;20(1):30-34.
(Continuing...)

- The highest percentage 'significant improvement' or 'cure' were for premenstrual syndrome (83%) and **migraine (83%)**

- Apart from these two, generally acute musculoskeletal presentations ,with mean duration of pain <u>less than 3 months</u> responded best.

- In my audit, the 'excellent+ good' improvement was seen mostly in **migraine (82%)** followed by knee pain (81%), and then fibromyalgia (80%)

- Among the 3 best improved diagnosis, 2 were with <u>chronic pain.</u>(fms, and migraine, <u>mean duration of pain 111 months, and 48 months respectively</u>)

An Audit of Acupuncture in a Single-Handed General Practice over One Year.
Anthony Stellon. ACUPUNCTURE IN MEDICINE 2001;19(1):36-42

- 140 patients

- (MYMOP) questionnaire ' measure yourself medical outcome profile' was used.

- Neck pain and Back pain were most common

- Mean duration of symptoms was 3 months (range 2 to 52 weeks)

- In my audit that was 31 months (more chronic pain)

- The mean number of acupuncture treatments was 4 (range 1 to 10), same as my audit.

An Audit of Acupuncture in a Single-Handed General Practice over One Year.
Anthony Stellon. ACUPUNCTURE IN MEDICINE 2001;19(1):36-42
(continuing..)

- 31% of patients had no effect, 31% were improved, and 38% were much improved.

- In my audit was 10% no effect, 41% improved, and 31% much improved

==➔ similar results except 'no effect group',

   which may be due to different measurement tools or difference in duration of symptoms.

An Audit of Acupuncture in a Single-Handed General Practice over One Year.
Anthony Stellon. ACUPUNCTURE IN MEDICINE 2001;19(1):36-42 (continuing..)

- In this audit, patients with symptoms of **shorter duration were more likely to benefit** from acupuncture treatment than those with more chronic symptoms(>12 weeks)

- The mean duration of pain in my audit was a lot longer(31 months versus 3), however non-healed patients were less.(10% versus 31%)

- In my audit **overall(1091 cases)**, there was no correlation between duration of symptoms and outcomes. (R: 0.026)

- However the **cases/diagnosis groups with best outcomes were having longer duration of pain** as complaint.

The best results (>50% improvement) In my audit were obtained in :

• 1st: *Migraine and tension headache 82%*
Mean duration of pain was 111 months

• 2nd: *Knee pain 81%*
Mean duration of pain was 19 months.

• 3rd :*Fibromyalgia and anxiety disorders 80%*
Mean duration of pain was 48 months.

 Overall mean duration of pain (of 1091 cases) was 31 months.

Which shows that the best results were obtained more among chronic pain patients.

- Therefore, ACUPUNCTURE (AP) can be considered as an encouraging treatment for chronic pain patients.

- *The UK NICE GUIDELINES 2020 (GID – NG10069) recommends that acupuncture be considered for chronic pain*

An Audit of the Effectiveness of Acupuncture on Musculoskeletal Pain in Primary Health
Care Elisa Kam, Guy Eslick, Ian Campbell.
ACUPUNCTURE IN MEDICINE 2002;20(1):35-38.

- From 92 patient records.

- Conditions treated:
- 23% backache; 18% neck pain, 13% shoulder pain, 8% headaches
  (similiar to my audit)

- The mean number of acupuncture treatments was 3 (in my audit was
  4.3)

- The benefit was based on the last recorded entry in the patient notes or
  calling the patients.

- The reported treatment benefit was 34% excellent, 35% good, and 31%
  poor. Success rate 35-69%

- *in my audit was 31% excellent,and 41% good, and 30% poor.*

Audit of Acupuncture to Stop Smoking
P A Cray. ACUPUNCTURE IN MEDICINE.May 1994 Vol 12

in this audit

- 10% of smokers stopped smoking.
- And 60% reduced the number of cigarettes.

So, if we define it in the same way as my audit, it makes 70% as success rate.

In my audit 90% of patients reduced the number of cigarettes per day by 80% and more.

In conclusion:

- This audit included a <u>large variety of patients(46 different diagnosis)</u> predominantly musculoskeletal pain, and a large number of cases (1091).

- Success rates (72-77%) were similiar to other audits, however the percentage of 'non responders' was less.(10%)

- The high success rate and few non-responders can be related to the <u>appropriate selection of patients</u> in the PMR clinic other than general primary care.

- The audit allowed me to see the diagnosis where acupuncture achieved the greatest success rates.

- Therefore it enabled me to advise and inform my patients for ;

- **which diagnosis acupuncture is most reliable,

- **even very few sessions may be enough for improvement,

- **and that they should not be pessimistic for the chronicity of their pain or for being elderly, since these were not negative factors for improvement.

Dr. Evren KUL PANZA